Table of Contents

Introduction

The high metabolism diet can be beneficial for weight loss, but more research needs to be done on its effectiveness and safety. By eating the right kinds of foods, you may be able to increase your metabolism and burn body fat as opposed to carbs, leading to weight loss. People with certain medical conditions should be careful about changing their diet. Low carb diets may help people with diabetes lose weight and control their blood sugar levels. Everyone on a high metabolic diet should be aware of the ketone levels in their body. This book contains all you need to know about metabolism diet.

Metabolic Diet

Whether you're looking to shed a few pounds or start a lifelong change, altering the way your body burns calories may be beneficial. New diets emerge based on the latest research. One of the latest diet trends is the metabolic diet, which aims to change how your body metabolizes food. The term "metabolic diet" includes diets such as the:

• fast metabolism diet

• high metabolism diet

• metabolism miracle

• MD diet factor

These diets are essentially a new spin on the Atkins diet, which emphasizes reducing your carbohydrate intake to lose weight. The big difference is that not all carbs are equal in the metabolic diet. Many versions of the metabolic diet include complex carbohydrates, such as whole grains, oats, and brown rice, but exclude refined carbs, such as processed breads, flours, and sugars. One component of these diets is to eat small meals throughout the day — typically three regular meals with two snacks — to help kick-start your metabolism. Frequent, small meals may help you manage hunger better throughout the day.

Changing Your Metabolism

Your body converts food into fuel. The faster your metabolism is, the faster your body can turn nutrients from food into energy. Having a slow metabolism means your body tends to store nutrients as fat instead of burning them up. A high metabolism diet aims to make your metabolism faster, so you burn fat instead of storing it. In low-carb diets, your body will shift to burning fat for energy, which leads to the production of compounds called ketones, which are thought to decrease appetite. The goal of these diets is to teach your body to burn body fat for energy. Ketones are acids made in the body when there isn't enough insulin to get sugar from your blood, and your body turns to burning fat instead of carbs. A buildup of too many ketones can be toxic, a condition called ketoacidosis. People with diabetes have to pay special attention to ketones. A small amount of ketones in your body is nothing to worry about. See your doctor if you have high ketone levels. Some of these diets promise weight loss of up to 20 pounds over four weeks. While there are many testimonials for these claims, studies are lacking. Most healthcare professionals consider such quick weight loss unsafe and unsustainable. There is also evidence that losing a significant amount of weight rapidly can slow your metabolism, which makes it easier to regain weight. In general, people with diabetes must take special care when dieting and pay special attention to their food intake and blood sugar levels. However, Source shows that low carb diets are beneficial for people with type 1 diabetes, as they can help reduce insulin doses and improve blood sugar control. Every person is different, so not all diets are right for everyone. People with specific medical conditions should be particularly wary of diets. Consult with your doctor before starting a metabolic-related diet or any other diet. Be sure to tell your doctor about any medical conditions or allergies you have. The overall goal of metabolic-centered diets is to create lasting changes in your diet and lifestyle. The amount of time you spend on the diet depends on how much weight you want to lose. After you lose the weight you intended to lose, there should be a stabilization period in which you get used to your new body and keep it at that target weight. Critics of these diets believe that anyone who goes on a diet will eventually go off of it and fall back into the habits that got them in trouble in the first place. This is why the metabolic diet is thought of more as a lifestyle change. In order to maintain your weight and not fall back into old habits, you will need to change what you eat and how you eat for good.

Fast Metabolism Diet

The Fast Metabolism Diet is a nutrition program that promises to help you lose up to 20 pounds (9 kg) in 28 days. It was developed by Haylie Pomroy, a celebrity nutritionist and wellness consultant with an academic background in animal science. The diet claims that eating particular foods at certain times tricks your metabolism into speeding up, resulting in weight loss. In addition to a weekly food plan, you receive an extensive list of foods to avoid. The diet also encourages exercise 2–3 times per week. If you haven't reached your goal weight by the end of the first 28-day cycle, you are encouraged to start again, staying on the diet until you have lost your desired amount of weight. Once you've reached your weight goal, you are told you can maintain your results by repeating one week of the cycle every month — or the full four-week cycle once every six months. Although some principles of this nutrition program are supported by science, most of its claims are not based on solid scientific evidence.

How To Follow The Fast Metabolism Diet

The Fast Metabolism Diet program is split into three phases which are repeated on a weekly basis for a total of four weeks. Each phase emphasizes different foods and provides recommendations for various physical activities. Portion sizes vary by phase and depending on the amount of weight you want to lose.

Phase 1 (Monday–Tuesday)

The diet's promoters claim that this phase unwinds stress and convinces your body that it is no longer trying to store fat. During these two days, you should eat a high-glycemic, carb-rich diet with moderate amounts of protein. Fats should be avoided. This is meant to reduce stress and anxiety, prepare your body for weight loss and encourage your adrenal glands to produce lower amounts of the stress hormone cortisol. Foods to eat include high-glycemic fruits, such as pears, mango, pineapple and cantaloupe, as well as high-carb whole grains, such as oatmeal, brown rice, spelt and brown-rice pasta. This phase also promotes foods rich in vitamins B and C, such as lean beef, lentils, oranges, turkey and kiwi. These are thought to stimulate your thyroid to burn fats, protein and carbs more efficiently — and convert sugar into energy instead of storing it as fat. During this phase, you are encouraged to include at least one aerobic workout.

Phase 2 (Wednesday–Thursday)

This phase is supposed to unlock fat stores and build muscle. During these two days, your diet should be rich in protein and non-starchy, alkalizing vegetables, yet low in carbs and fats. Lean, high-protein foods that help create muscle include beef, bison, turkey, fish and chicken. This phase also includes vegetables, such as cabbage, broccoli, kale, spinach, cucumbers and collard greens. The diet plan claims that these vegetables are alkalizing and supposedly lower the acidity of your blood, stimulating your liver to release fat cells. At the same time, they're said to provide the enzymes and phytonutrients needed to break down high-protein foods. However, keep in mind that your body tightly regulates your blood pH level, keeping it slightly alkaline around 7.36–7.44. In fact, it would have detrimental consequences if the pH of your blood fell out of its normal range. So, while the vegetables promoted for the second phase are very healthy, they're not healthy because of their supposed effects on blood pH. During the second phase, you are encouraged to do at least one weight-lifting session.

Phase 3 (Friday–Sunday)

This phase is designed to accelerate your metabolism and fat burning. During these three days, you are encouraged to add many healthy fats to your meals and snacks while consuming moderate amounts of protein and carbs. Foods to eat in this phase include olive or grapeseed oil, safflower mayonnaise, eggs, nuts, seeds, coconut, avocados and olives. Foods like seaweed, coconut oil, shrimp and lobster should also be included since the diet claims that they boost metabolism by stimulating your thyroid gland. During this phase, you are encouraged to pick an activity that allows you to unwind, such as yoga, meditation or even a massage. This is meant to lower stress hormone levels and increase the circulation of fat-burning compounds.

Certain foods can increase your metabolism. The higher your metabolism, the more calories you burn and the easier it is to maintain your weight or get rid of unwanted body fat. Here are foods that rev up your metabolism, which may help you lose weight.

Protein-Rich Foods

Protein-rich foods, such as meat, fish, eggs, dairy, legumes, nuts and seeds, could help increase your metabolism for a few hours. They do so by requiring your body to use more energy to digest them. This is known as the thermic effect of food (TEF). The TEF refers to the number of calories needed by your body to digest, absorb and process the nutrients in your meals. Research shows that protein-rich foods increase TEF the most. For example, they increase your metabolic rate by 15–30%, compared to 5–10% for carbs and 0–3% for fats. Protein-rich diets also reduce the drop in metabolism often seen during weight loss by helping your body hold on to its muscle mass. What's more, protein may also help keep you fuller for longer, which can prevent overeating.

Iron, Zinc and Selenium-Rich Foods

Iron, zinc and selenium each play different but equally important roles in the proper function of your body. However, they do have one thing in common: all three are required for the proper function of your thyroid gland, which regulates your metabolism. Research shows that a diet too low in iron, zinc or selenium may reduce the ability of your thyroid gland to produce sufficient amounts of hormones. This can slow down your metabolism. To help your thyroid function to the best of its ability, include zinc, selenium and iron-rich foods like meat, seafood, legumes, nuts and seeds in your daily menu.

Chili Peppers

Capsaicin, a chemical found in chili peppers, may boost your metabolism by increasing the number of calories and fat you burn. In fact, a review of 20 research studies reports that capsaicin can help your body burn around 50 extra calories per day. This effect was initially observed after taking 135–150 mg of capsaicin per day, but some studies report similar benefits with doses as low as 9–10 mg per day. Moreover, capsaicin may have appetite-reducing properties. According to a recent study, consuming 2 mg of capsaicin directly before each meal seems to reduce the number of calories consumed, especially from carbs. That said, not all studies agree on capsaicin's metabolism-boosting abilities.

Coffee

Studies report that the caffeine found in coffee can help increase metabolic rate by up to 11%. In fact, six different studies found that people who consume at least 270 mg of caffeine daily, or the equivalent of about three cups of coffee, burn an extra 100 calories per day. Furthermore, caffeine may also help your body burn fat for energy and seems especially effective at boosting your workout performance. However, its effects seem to vary from person to person, based on individual characteristics such as body weight and age.

Tea

According to research, the combination of caffeine and catechins that's found in tea may work to boost your metabolism. In particular, both oolong and green tea may increase metabolism by 4–10%. This could add up to burning an extra 100 calories per day. In addition, oolong and green teas may help your body use stored fat for energy more effectively, increasing your fat-burning ability by up to 17%. Nevertheless, as is the case with coffee, effects may vary from person to person.

Legumes and Pulses

Legumes and pulses, such as lentils, peas, chickpeas, beans and peanuts, are particularly high in protein compared to other plant foods. Studies suggest that their high protein content requires your body to burn a greater number of calories to digest them, compared to lower-protein foods. Legumes also contain a good amount of dietary fiber, such as resistant starch and soluble fiber, which your body can use to feed the good bacteria living in your intestines. In turn, these friendly bacteria produce short-chain fatty acids, which may help your body use stored fat as energy and maintain normal blood sugar levels. In one study, humans consuming a legume-rich diet for eight weeks experienced beneficial changes in metabolism and lost 1.5 times more weight than the control group. Legumes are also high in arginine, an amino acid that may increase the amount of carbs and fat your body can burn for energy. In addition, peas, faba beans and lentils also contain substantial amounts of the amino acid glutamine, which may help increase the number of calories burned during digestion.

Metabolism-Boosting Spices

Certain spices are thought to have particularly beneficial metabolism-boosting properties. For instance, research shows that dissolving 2 grams of ginger powder in hot water and drinking it with a meal may help you burn up to 43 more calories than drinking hot water alone. This hot ginger drink also seems to decrease levels of hunger and enhance feelings of satiety. Grains of paradise, another spice in the ginger family, may have similar effects. A recent study reported that participants given a 40-mg extract of grains of paradise burned 43 more calories in the following two hours than those given a placebo. That said, researchers also noted that part of the participants were non-responders, so the effects may vary from one person to another. Similarly, adding cayenne pepper to your meal may increase the amount of fat your body burns for energy, especially following a high-fat meal.

However, this fat-burning effect may only apply to people unaccustomed to consuming spicy foods.

Cacao

Cacao and cocoa are tasty treats that may also benefit your metabolism. For instance, studies in mice found that cocoa and cocoa extracts may promote the expression of genes that stimulate the use of fat for energy. This seems especially true in mice fed high-fat or high-calorie diets. Interestingly, one study suggests that cocoa may prevent the action of enzymes necessary to break down fat and carbs during digestion. In doing so, cocoa could theoretically play a role in preventing weight gain by reducing the absorption of some calories. However, human studies examining the effects of cocoa, cacao or cacao products such as dark chocolate are rare. More studies are needed before strong conclusions can be made. If you'd like to give cacao a try, opt for raw versions, as processing tends to reduce the amounts of beneficial compounds.

Apple Cider Vinegar

Apple cider vinegar may increase your metabolism. Several animal studies have shown vinegar to be particularly helpful in increasing the amount of fat burned for energy. In one study, mice given vinegar experienced an increase in the AMPK enzyme, which prompts the body to decrease fat storage and increase fat burning. In another study, obese rats treated with vinegar experienced an increase in the expression of certain genes, leading to reduced liver fat and belly fat storage. Apple cider vinegar is often claimed to boost metabolism in humans, but few studies have investigated the matter directly. Nevertheless, apple cider vinegar may still help you lose weight in other ways, such as slowing stomach emptying and enhancing feelings of fullness. One study in humans even showed that participants given four teaspoons (20 ml) of apple cider vinegar ate up to 275 fewer calories over the rest of the day. If you'd like to give apple cider vinegar a try, be careful to limit your daily consumption to two tablespoons (30 ml).

Coconut Oil

Coconut oil is experiencing a surge in popularity. That may be partly because coconut oil is high in medium-chain triglycerides (MCTs). This is contrary to most other types of fats, which usually contain higher amounts of long-chain fatty acids. Unlike long-chain fats, once MCTs are absorbed, they go directly to the liver to be turned into energy. This makes them less likely to be stored as fat. Interestingly, several studies show that MCTs can increase metabolic rate more than longer-chain fats. In addition, researchers report that a daily intake of 30 ml of coconut oil may successfully reduce waist size in obese individuals.

Water

Drinking enough water is a great way to stay hydrated. Additionally, it seems that drinking water may also temporarily boost metabolism by 24–30%. Researchers note that about 40% of that increase is explained by the additional calories needed to heat the water to body temperature. Yet, the effects only seem to last for 60–90 minutes after drinking it and may vary from one person to another.

Seaweed

Seaweed is a great source of iodine, a mineral required for the production of thyroid hormones and proper function of your thyroid gland. Thyroid hormones have various functions, one of which is to regulate your metabolic rate. Regularly consuming seaweed can help you meet your iodine needs and keep your metabolism running at a high rate. The reference daily intake of iodine for adults is 150 mcg per day. This can be met by consuming several servings of seaweed per week. Although, some types of seaweed such as kelp are extremely high in iodine and should not be consumed in large amounts. Fucoxanthin is another compound found in some varieties of seaweed that may help with metabolism. It's primarily found in brown seaweed varieties and may have anti-obesity effects by increasing the amount of calories you burn.

Foods To Avoid

The Fast Metabolism Diet warns against some foods which should be avoided whenever possible. These include:

• Wheat

• Corn

• Dairy

• Soy

• Dried fruit

• Fruit juices

• Refined sugar

• Artificial sweeteners and foods containing them

• Caffeine

• Alcohol

• Fat-free diet foods

However, the diet's founder does make an exception for vegetarians and vegans, who are allowed to eat three soy foods: tempeh, tofu and edamame. Note that these must be organic and not genetically modified (non-GMO). On this diet, non-organic produce and nitrate-containing meats are also banned because the additives, preservatives, pesticides, insecticides and hormones they may host are thought to slow down your liver's burning of fat.

Sample Menu

Here is a sample menu for the Fast Metabolism Diet, organized by phase. Keep in mind that portion sizes will depend on the phase and your personal weight loss goals.

Phase 1

- Breakfast: Dairy-free frozen mango smoothie
- Snack: Pineapple
- Lunch: Grilled chicken breast and wild rice
- Snack: Strawberries
- Dinner: Grilled fish with vegetables
- Snack: Watermelon

Phase 2

- Breakfast: Egg white, spinach and mushroom omelet
- Snack: Turkey jerky
- Lunch: Chicken and vegetable soup
- Snack: Smoked salmon and cucumbers
- Dinner: Grilled lean-cut lamb satay
- Snack: A glass of unsweetened almond milk

- Breakfast: Toast topped with egg, tomato and onion
- Snack: Celery with almond butter
- Lunch: Spinach, tomato and chicken salad
- Snack: Cucumber dipped in homemade guacamole
- Dinner: Shrimp with spinach fettuccine
- Snack: Walnuts

A Few Additional Rules

Aside from following the diet and physical activity guidelines for each phase, the Fast Metabolism Diet includes a few additional rules.

- Eat five times per day.
- Eat every 3–4 hours except when sleeping.
- Eat within 30 minutes of waking.
- Follow the phases in order.
- Stick to the foods allowed in each phase.
- Exercise according to the phase you're in.
- Drink half of your body weight (measured in pounds) in ounces of water each day.

• Avoid wheat, corn, soy, dairy, dried fruit, fruit juices, refined sugar, artificial sweeteners, caffeine, alcohol and fat-free diet foods.

• Eat organic whenever possible.

• Ensure that meats are nitrate-free.

• Follow the plan for the full 28 days and repeat until your weight loss goal is achieved.

• Repeat the fast metabolism plan for a full 28 days every six months or for one week every month.

Fast Metabolism Diet And Weight Loss

The Fast Metabolism Diet likely helps you lose weight for several reasons. First, it incorporates plenty of whole foods. This may increase your fiber intake, which may contribute to weight loss. Next, excluding soy, wheat, refined sugar and sweeteners further cuts out many processed foods from your diet. This can naturally reduce the number of calories consumed, further promoting weight loss. What's more, the prescribed weekly physical exercise is likely to increase the number of calories burned, further contributing to the energy deficit needed for weight loss. Moreover, hydration — emphasized strongly in the diet — can lower appetite and may help you burn a few more calories to promote additional weight loss.

Other Benefits Fast Metabolism Diet

The Fast Metabolism Diet may offer additional benefits. By incorporating plenty of fruits, vegetables, lean protein and healthy fats, it's richer in vitamins and minerals than some other diet plans. Its extensive list of foods to avoid also naturally curbs your intake of highly processed, empty-calorie foods, leaving more room for nutrient-rich ones. The fiber content may also promote gut health, blood sugar control and immune and brain function.

Potential Downsides

The Fast Metabolism Diet has major drawbacks as well. Here are some of the most prominent.

Based on Pseudoscience

The Fast Metabolism Diet puts a strong emphasis on consuming specific foods in a certain order to boost metabolism and promote weight loss.However, there is little scientific evidence backing such principles. For instance, Phase 1 advocates a high-glycemic, carb-rich diet as a way to encourage your adrenal glands to produce fewer stress hormones and prepare your body for weight loss. However, research shows that high intake of simple carbs may raise stress hormone levels — not diminish them. Despite claims to the contrary, there is also no evidence that eating carb-rich foods for two days in a row will reduce stress and anxiety — or gird you for weight loss. Phase 2 advocates for a high intake of protein and supposedly alkalizing vegetables as a way to build muscle, keep your pH in balance and help your liver release fat cells from storage. High-protein diets are indeed linked to building muscle, especially when combined with resistance training. However, there is no evidence that vegetables are effective at treating an imbalanced blood pH. In fact, there is ample evidence that your body can naturally maintain blood pH within a strict range — regardless of what you eat.Furthermore, no studies suggest that alkalizing vegetables can stimulate your liver to release fat cells from storage. Another main principle of the diet is that it will keep your metabolism stimulated, which will get it to work faster and burn more weight.However, there is absolutely no research to support this theory of "surprising" your metabolism as a way to lose more weight. Though some foods can cause slight increases in metabolism, any increase is minor and unlikely to help you lose a substantial amount of weight. Finally, there is no evidence that this diet's emphasis on organic foods and nitrate-free meats has any boosting effect on your liver's ability to burn fat.

May Be Unsustainable

The Fast Metabolism Diet is frequently criticized for being unsustainable.Many people complain that it requires too much measuring, weighing and food prepping to fit into a busy lifestyle.Such a specific and restrictive diet may also be difficult to follow if you eat out regularly or attend barbecues, birthday parties or holiday events.

Restricts Some Beneficial Foods

Although the long list of foods to avoid does cull many processed foods from people's diets, it also cuts out some beneficial ones.For instance, soy is linked to a modest decrease in cholesterol levels and may also contain some cancer-fighting compounds. Caffeine is another banned food on this diet which is associated with improved brain function, protection against Alzheimer's and Parkinson's and a lower likelihood of depression.

Recipes

Peanut Butter Pops

Ingredients

- 3 large bananas
- 6 pop sticks
- 6 tablespoons crunchy peanut butter

If you are not a fan of peanut butter, use healthy Nutella instead. Nutella is a hazelnut-based food product with a consistency similar to that of smooth peanut butter.

Directions

• Peel and cut bananas in half lengthwise.

• Press popsicle sticks gently onto flat side of each banana slice.

• Freeze bananas on wax paper for 30 minutes.

• Remove from freezer and spread one tablespoon of peanut butter on each banana. Serve immediately or refreeze.

Quick Pick-Me-Up Trail Mix

Ingredients

• 4 cups air-popped popcorn

• 4 tablespoons raisins

• 4 tablespoons unsalted peanuts

On its own, popcorn doesn't add much to your metabolism but, when combined, with nutrient-rich raisins and peanuts, as it is here, the fiber helps move carbohydrates and fats through your digestive system. Other great trail mix combinations are almonds, pistachios, sunflower seeds, and dried fruits such as apricots, bananas, and cranberries.

Direction

• Pop popcorn with an air popper.

• Combine popcorn with raisins and nuts.

Sugar-Free Lemonade Bars

Makes 8 8-ounce servings

Ingredients

• Crystal Light lemonade drink mix

• ¼ cup minced fresh mint leaves

• Water

• Popsicle sticks

Directions

Although these lemonade bars don't provide tons of nutrients, they are naturally sugar-free and very low calorie. Keep them on hand for a quick snack in between meals to help prevent the overeating that leads to a slower metabolism. They are also perfect for a late-night snack as they are caffeine free.

• Make your favorite Crystal Light drink as directed and mix in fresh mint leaves.

• Pour beverage into ice cube trays or other bar molds. Add popsicle sticks.

• Freeze for 1 hour or more.

Serves 12

Ingredients

• Nonstick cooking spray

• 2 cups all-purpose flour

• cup unsweetened cocoa powder

• 1 teaspoon baking soda

• ½ teaspoon sea salt

• 1 cup sugar

• 2 tablespoons canola oil

• 1 egg white

• 1 cup nonfat vanilla yogurt

• 2 teaspoons vanilla extract

• ¼ cup fat-free fudge topping or chocolate syrup

Directions

Spicy cocoa, nutrient-rich yogurt, and naturally low-fat egg white make this dessert more easily digestible. Feel free to add a few fresh raspberries, strawberries, or even mandarin oranges for added nutrition and fruity texture.

• Preheat oven to 350°F. Spray 8-inch-square pan with light cooking spray. Set aside.

• In a large bowl, mix the flour, cocoa, baking soda, salt, and sugar well.

• In a medium bowl, thoroughly mix the oil, egg white, yogurt, vanilla, and fudge topping. Add the wet mixture to the dry mixture and mix thoroughly.

• Pour the batter into the prepared baking dish and bake for 35 minutes.

New York Cheesecake With Wild Berries

Serves 8

Ingredients

• 1 cup reduced-fat graham crackers, finely crushed

• ¼ cup butter, melted

• 16 ounces fat-free cream cheese

• ¼ cup sugar substitute such as Splenda

• 1 teaspoon vanilla extract

• 2 egg whites

• 3 tablespoons cake flour

• ¼ teaspoon sea salt

• ½ cup fat-free milk

• 1 cup fresh wild berries such as blackberries, raspberries, or blueberries, for garnish

Directions

Sugar substitutes save on calories and don't cause fluctuations in your blood glucose as regular sugar does.

• Preheat oven to 350°F. Stir the graham cracker crumbs and butter together until they are evenly mixed. Press crumb mixture into the bottom of a baking dish.

• Mix cream cheese, sugar substitute, vanilla, and egg whites in a standing mixer or medium bowl with hand mixer. Add the cake flour, salt, and milk. Mix thoroughly. Pour batter into the crust. Bake for 1 hour. Cool about 10 minutes before placing in fridge. Refrigerate at least 3 hours before serving. Serve with fresh wild berries.

Chocolate Cupcakes

Serves 12

• 1 cup self-rising flour

• ½ cup nonfat dried milk powder

• 1 3.4-ounce box sugar-free chocolate Jell-O pudding mix

• 1 tablespoon unsweetened cocoa powder

• ¼ cup sugar substitute such as Splenda

- 1 teaspoon vanilla extract
- ½ cup applesauce
- ¼ teaspoon baking soda
- 4 egg whites
- Pinch sea salt

Directions

Nonfat milk powder is as high in protein and calcium as liquid milk and is naturally fat free. It's a natural milk substitute and can be used in many recipes.

- Preheat oven to 350°F. Mix flour, milk powder, Jell-O mix, cocoa, and sugar substitute in a medium bowl. In a separate bowl, blend the vanilla, applesauce, and baking soda.

- In a small bowl, beat the egg whites and salt until stiff. Add the flour mixture to the egg whites, beating with an electric mixer. Add the applesauce and beat until blended.

- Line a muffin tin with paper cupcake wrappers and fill each ¾ of the way with batter. Bake for 20 minutes or until toothpick inserted comes out clean.

BURN IT UP

Chocolate is good for you. Well, sort of. It's still high in calories, but an ounce of dark chocolate will provide you with antioxidants and may help lower your blood pressure. Just keep in mind that the darker the chocolate, the better off you are because dark chocolate contains the highest amount of flavonoids.

Serves 16

Ingredients

- Unsalted butter for greasing pan
- 1 cup nonfat sour cream
- ½ cup sugar
- ½ cup brown sugar
- 2 eggs
- 2 teaspoons vanilla extract
- 1¾ cups flour
- 1 teaspoon baking powder
- 1 teaspoon baking soda
- ¼ teaspoon sea salt
- ¼ teaspoon ground nutmeg

Directions

Nutmeg possesses antioxidant and immunomodulatory properties, making it a welcome addition to many desserts.

• Preheat oven to 350°F. Grease 9" × 13" pan with unsalted butter and set aside.

• In a large bowl, combine sour cream and sugar; beat well. Add brown sugar and beat. Add eggs, one at a time, beating well after each addition. Stir in vanilla.

• Sift flour with baking powder, baking soda, salt, and nutmeg. Stir into sour cream mixture and beat at medium speed for 1 minute. Pour into prepared pan.

• Bake for 25–35 minutes or until cake pulls away from sides of pan and top springs back when touched lightly in center. Cool completely on wire rack; store covered at room temperature.

Citrus-Glazed Grilled Pineapple

Serves 4

Ingredients

• 4 thick slices pineapple, about 1-inch each

• Juice of ½ lime

• Juice of ½ orange

• 4 teaspoons brown sugar

Directions

The nutrients in grilled pineapple are accented by the citric acid, found in the lime and orange, which works to metabolize the natural brown sugar.

• Preheat grill. In small bowl, combine lime and orange juices. Brush both sides of the pineapple slices with juice and sprinkle with brown sugar. Place pineapple slices on a hot grill; turn after 3 minutes. Grill another 3 minutes.

• When the pineapples are done, you should have a nice brown caramel color.

Honey-Glazed Nectarines With Citrus Mascarpone

Serves 2

Ingredients

• 2 nectarines, cut in halves, pits discarded

• 4 teaspoons mascarpone cheese

• ½ teaspoon finely grated lemon zest

• ½ teaspoon finely grated orange zest

• 2 tablespoons honey

Directions

Nectarines have natural sugars and potassium and are a good source of lycopene.

• Place the nectarines, cut side down on a hot grill for 5 minutes.

• In small mixing bowl, mix mascarpone with lemon and orange zest. Spoon mixture into the center of nectarines. Drizzle with honey and serve.

Sour Cream Coffee Cake

Serves 20

Ingredients

• Nonstick cooking spray

• 1½ cups flour

• ¾ cup packed light brown sugar

• ½ teaspoon baking powder

• 1 teaspoon baking soda

• 1 teaspoon ground cinnamon

• 1 teaspoon sea salt

• ¾ cup fat-free sour cream

• 2 tablespoons canola oil

• 1 cup unsweetened applesauce

Directions

Because of its natural sweetness, high fiber content, and good amount of vitamin C, applesauce is one of the best substitutes for sugar in dessert recipes.It helps keep carbs down, while bringing flavor and food-digesting fiber up.

• Preheat oven to 350°F. Coat a square baking pan with light cooking spray.

• Mix the flour, brown sugar, baking powder, baking soda, cinnamon, and salt in a large bowl.

• Separately, mix the sour cream, oil, and applesauce in a small bowl. Add sour cream mixture to flour mixture. Mix well but do not beat.

• Pour batter into cake pan and bake until done, about 40 minutes, or until toothpick inserted comes out clean.

Baked Peach Apple Crumble

Serves 4

Ingredients

• Nonstick cooking spray

• 2 tart apples, peeled, cored, and sliced

• 4 medium peaches, blanched, skins and pits removed, sliced

- Juice of ½ lemon
- ½ cup flour
- ¼ cup dark brown sugar
- ½ teaspoon cinnamon
- ½ teaspoon coriander seed, ground
- ½ teaspoon cardamom seed, ground
- ½ teaspoon sea salt
- 1 cup oatmeal
- ½ stick butter, softened

Directions

You should use spices whenever you can. The cinnamon, coriander, and cardamom in this recipe boost your metabolism instantaneously.

- Preheat the oven to 350 °F. Prepare a gratin dish or baking dish with nonstick spray.
- Distribute the apple and peach slices in the dish and sprinkle with lemon juice.
- Using your hands, thoroughly mix together the flour, brown sugar, spices, salt, oatmeal, and butter. Spread over the crisp and bake for 45 minutes, or until the fruit is bubbling and the top is brown.
- Serve with vanilla ice cream or whipped cream.

BURN IT UP

Oatmeal is a marvelous choice for healthy fiber, both soluble and insoluble. The insoluble fiber found in oatmeal is good for people with diabetes because it slows down the digestion of starch, preventing a sharp rise in blood glucose levels after a meal. Soluble fiber aids in the processing and elimination of food, moving it quickly and efficiently through your body. The fiber in oatmeal also has cancer-fighting qualities and may reduce LDL cholesterol levels.

Baked Stuffed Apples

Serves 2

Ingredients

• 2 large apples, such as Macintosh, Rome, or Granny Smith

• 2 teaspoons brown sugar

• ½ teaspoon cinnamon

• 2 teaspoons chopped walnuts

• 2 teaspoons raisins

• 2 teaspoons butter

Directions

Baked apples are high in fiber and vitamin C. They are a great way to enjoy a lower-fat, lower-calorie dessert that still has plenty of flavor.

• Preheat the oven to 350 °F. Using a corer, remove the center portions of the apples, being careful not to cut through the bottom of the apple.

• Form a cup with a double layer of aluminum foil, going of the way up the apple. This will stabilize the apple when baking.

• Mix together the brown sugar, cinnamon, walnuts, and raisins and stuff the mixture into the apples. Top each apple with 1 teaspoon of butter. Put 1 tablespoon of water into the aluminum foil cups.

• Bake for 25 minutes, or until the apples are soft when pricked with a fork.

BURN IT UP

Apples are fabulous for you—and your metabolism. The active ingredient in apple pulp is pectin, a soluble form of fiber that helps reduce LDL ("bad") cholesterol by keeping it in the intestinal tract until it is eliminated. Pectin also creates a sensation of fullness and suppresses appetite. A study published in the Journal of the National Cancer Institute shows that pectin binds certain cancer-causing compounds in the colon, accelerating their removal from the body.

Ricotta Tort With Candied Orange

Serves 6–8

Ingredients

- 5 eggs
- 1-pound skim milk ricotta cheese
- 4 ounces nonfat cream cheese
- 1 teaspoon vanilla extract
- 1 teaspoon salt
- ¾ cup candied orange peel, chopped
- 1 cup chocolate chips or chopped chocolate pieces
- Nonstick cooking spray

Directions

Ricotta cheese is rich in calcium, vitamin A, and iron, and is a great source of protein.

- Preheat oven to 350°F. Separate the eggs and beat the whites until stiff. Set aside.
- Put the yolks, cheeses, vanilla, and salt in the food processor and whirl until smooth.

• Place in a bowl and fold in the egg whites, the orange peel, and the chocolate bits. Prepare a pie dish with nonstick spray. Pour in the egg mixture and bake for 45 minutes or until set and golden on top.

Carrot Cake With Ginger

Serves 8–10

Ingredients

• 4 eggs, separated

• ½ cup brown sugar

• 1½ cups grated carrots

• 1 tablespoon lemon juice

• Fine zest of ½ fresh orange

• ½ cup corn flour

• 1-inch fresh gingerroot, peeled and minced

• 1½ teaspoons baking soda

• ½ teaspoon sea salt

Directions

This cake is a triple threat: carrots are great for your eyesight, ginger root is great for boosting your metabolic rate, and corn flour is higher in fiber and potassium than traditional flour. Add all that up and you've got a more body-efficient—and metabolism-boosting— carrot cake than found in other recipes.

• Butter a springform pan and preheat oven to 325°F. Beat the egg whites until stiff and set aside.

• Beat the egg yolks, brown sugar, and carrots together. Add lemon juice, orange zest, and corn flour. When smooth, add the gingerroot, baking soda, and salt. Gently fold in the egg whites.

• Pour the cake batter into the springform pan and bake for 1 hour or until done, when toothpick inserted comes out clean.

Chocolate Meringue With Hazelnuts

Makes about 40 cookies

Ingredients

• ½ cup sugar, divided

• ¼ cup unsweetened cocoa powder

• teaspoon sea salt

• 3 egg whites (from extra-large eggs)

• teaspoon cream of tartar

• ½ cup hazelnuts, lightly toasted, skinned, and coarsely chopped

Directions

Most of the fat in this recipe comes from the nuts. If you're not a fan of hazelnuts, you can sub in alternatives like pistachios or walnuts.

• Preheat oven to 275°F. Line two cookie sheets with parchment paper. Sift ¼ cup of sugar and ¼ cup of cocoa powder together in a bowl. Add salt.

• Beat egg whites with cream of tartar. When peaks begin to form, add the remaining ¼ cup sugar, a teaspoon at a time. Slowly beat in the cocoa mixture. The meringue should be stiff and shiny.

• Add chopped nuts. Drop by the teaspoonful on the parchment paper. Bake for 45–50 minutes. Cool on baking sheets. Serve or place in an airtight container for later use.

BURN IT UP

Because the hours between lunch and dinner can create a mini-fast, many crave sweets in the late afternoon. Before you reach for a candy bar, a piece of chocolate, or a brownie, seek out snacks that contain all three macronutrients—like carbohydrates, protein, and fat. Hazelnuts will provide you with all three!

Serves 4

Ingredients

• 2 squares bittersweet chocolate

• ½ cup sugar

• 1 tablespoon butter plus 1 tablespoon for soufflé dish

• 2 tablespoons raspberry liqueur like Chambord

• 3 tablespoons rice flour or cornstarch

• 3 tablespoons cold reduced-fat milk

• 4 egg yolks

• 5 egg whites

• Pinch cream of tartar

• ½ pint fresh raspberries

Directions

Berries in general are fiber and antioxidant rich, so add a few blackberries to this recipe, if desired, for extra flavor, color, and texture.

• Preheat the oven to 375°F. In a medium-sized, heavy saucepan, melt the chocolate with the sugar, butter, and liqueur. Remove from heat. Whisk the flour and milk together and add to the chocolate mixture.

• Beat the egg yolks, one at a time, into the chocolate mixture. Whip the egg whites and cream of tartar together until stiff. Fold the egg whites into the chocolate mixture and pour into a buttered 1½-quart soufflé dish.

• Bake for 35–40 minutes or until puffed and brown. Pour fresh raspberries over each portion and garnish with whipped cream if desired.

Baked Espresso Crème

Serves 4

Ingredients

• 3 tablespoons instant espresso powder

• 2 tablespoons boiling water

• 1½ cups whipping cream

• 3 whole eggs

• 4 teaspoons cornstarch

• 4 teaspoons cold water

• ½ cup sugar, or to taste

• 1 teaspoon vanilla extract

Directions

Coffee may improve brain function and has been linked to lowering the risk for diabetes and certain cancers. Caffeine also naturally stimulates your metabolism.

• Preheat oven to 325°F. Whisk together the espresso powder and boiling water, add the cream, and beat in the eggs. Whisk the cornstarch and water together until smooth and beat into the mixture.

• Add the rest of the ingredients and stir well. Place 4 buttered 6-ounce custard cups in a roasting pan of hot water in the middle of the oven. Add the custard.

• Bake for 50–60 minutes. Serve warm, at room temperature, or chilled with whipped cream.

Zesty Lime Pie

Serves: 8

Ingredients

Crust:

• 15 graham crackers, crushed

• 2 tablespoons butter, melted

Filling:

- cup frozen apple juice concentrate, thawed
- 1 envelope unflavored gelatin
- ½ cup sugar
- 1 tablespoon grated lime zest
- cup lime juice
- 1 teaspoon pure vanilla extract
- 1½ cups plain low-fat yogurt

Directions

Lime juice is well known as a cure for scurvy, a disease caused by lack of vitamin C. The flavonoids found in limes have antioxidant and anticancer properties as well.

- To make the crust, mix together the graham cracker crumbs and butter in a bowl. Grease a 9-inch pie pan. Transfer the crumb mixture to the prepared pan and pat onto the bottom and sides, forming an even layer. Place in the freezer.

- To make the filling, pour the apple juice concentrate into a saucepan, add the gelatin, and let the mixture stand for a few minutes to allow the gelatin to soften. Stir in the sugar and heat the mixture over low heat until the gelatin and sugar dissolve. Pour into a bowl and add 2 teaspoons of the lime zest, the lime juice, and the vanilla. Place the mixture in the refrigerator until partially set (the consistency of unbeaten egg whites), about 30 minutes.

• In standing mixer or with hand mixer, whip the lime mixture until fluffy. Add the yogurt and whip again. Remove the crust from the freezer and pour the lime mixture into it. Sprinkle the remaining 1 teaspoon lime zest over the top. Chill the pie until firm before serving.

BURN IT UP

Yogurt is an excellent source of calcium that also provides about 9 grams of animal protein per 6-ounce serving. It also has a good supply of riboflavin, vitamin B12, potassium, and magnesium. One of the most beneficial aspects of yogurt comes from the use of active, good bacteria, known as probiotics, that adjust the natural balance of organisms, known as microflora, in the intestines to aid digestion.

Serves: 4

Ingredients

• 4 pears, peeled, cored, and halved lengthwise

• 2 cups cranberry juice

• 2 tablespoons sugar

• ½ teaspoon ground cinnamon

• ½ teaspoon ground cloves

• 1 teaspoon grated orange zest

• 1 teaspoon grated lemon zest

Directions

Pears are a nutritious fruit that are naturally high in fiber and antioxidants. The high amounts of pectin found in pears aids in digestion and promotes healthy cholesterol levels. They have a low glycemic index, meaning they produce a more gradual rise in blood sugar and insulin levels.

• Combine all the ingredients in a saucepan.

• Bring to a boil, cover, reduce the heat to low, and simmer until tender, about 15 minutes. Serve the pears warm or chilled.

Serves: 4

Ingredients

• 2 tablespoons sugar

• teaspoon sea salt

• 1 cup nonfat milk

• ¼ teaspoon pure vanilla extract

• 2–3 teaspoons sherry

• 3 egg whites, lightly beaten

• Spiced Cherry Sauce:

• 1 8-ounce can cherries, unsweetened or fresh, pitted

• 3 drops of red food coloring

• 1 teaspoon cornstarch

• 2 teaspoons water or lemon juice

• Pinch ground cloves

• Pinch ground cinnamon

• Pinch ground ginger

Directions

Fresh cherries are a fiber-filled, natural source of vitamin A, and studies have shown that they may reduce the risk for heart disease, diabetes, and certain cancers.

• Preheat oven to 325 °F. In a saucepan, combine the sugar, salt, and milk. Place over medium heat and stir until the sugar dissolves. Cool. Add the vanilla, sherry, and egg whites. Stir well and pour through a sieve into a 2-cup baking dish. Place in a baking pan, and pour hot water into the pan to reach halfway up the sides of the dish. Bake until a knife comes out clean, about 1 hour.

• Meanwhile, make the sauce: in a saucepan, combine the cherries and food coloring. Place over medium heat and bring to a simmer. In a small bowl, stir together the cornstarch and water or lemon juice. Add to the pan and cook, stirring, until the sauce is clear, about 5 minutes. Stir in the spices.

• Remove the custard from the oven. Serve warm with the warm cherry sauce drizzled over the top.

Chocolate Banana Cake

Serves 9

Ingredients

- ¾ cup whole wheat flour

- ¾ cup all-purpose flour

- 1 teaspoon baking powder

- ¼ teaspoon baking soda

- ¾ cup sugar substitute such as Splenda

- teaspoon salt

- ⅔ cup dark chocolate chips

- ⅔ cup mashed ripe bananas

- cup unsweetened applesauce

- cup fat-free plain yogurt

- ½ cup Egg Beaters

- 1 teaspoon banana extract

Directions

This dessert is remarkably high in nutritional value thanks to the high fiber from the wheat flour, the protein from the yogurt and Egg Beaters, and the antioxidant-rich dark chocolate.

- Preheat oven to 350 °F.

- Combine flours, baking powder, baking soda, Splenda, salt, and chocolate chips in a large bowl and stir well. Add remaining ingredients; stir until smooth.

• Pour batter into an 8-inch-square pan. Bake for 30 minutes. Cool and cut into nine squares.

Chocolate Chunk Brownies

Serves 12

Ingredients

• Nonstick cooking spray

• 1 box Betty Crocker Hershey's Triple Chunk Supreme Brownie Mix

• 2 ounces dark chocolate chips

• ½ cup Egg Beaters

• ½ cup sugar-free chocolate syrup

• 3 tablespoons water

Directions

Often enhanced with additional nutrients, Egg Beaters is a reputable egg substitute that consists mainly of egg whites. Egg Beaters is also cholesterol free.

• Coat a 9" × 13" baking dish with nonstick spray.

• Stir brownie mix, dark chocolate chips, Egg Beaters, syrup, and water together in a bowl. Blend well. Pour mix into baking dish.

• Bake in oven at 350°F for 26–28 minutes.